Engaging Dementia Activities

Fostering Relationships via Interactive Play, Enjoyable Games, Mind Challenging Puzzles to Boost Memory and Build Trust with Your Loved One

Dear Caregivers,

We have heard your questions, understand your struggles, and we see that for a long time, many of you have been wondering, "What can I do? What can they do? What can we do together?"

To help resolve this issue, we have created a unique activity book designed for individuals with cognitive disabilities.

This covers everyone experiencing a cognitive decline, such as Dementia or Alzheimer's, perhaps those learning to communicate again after a stroke or traumatic brain injury, or those living with a degenerative disease. The contents of this activity book include puzzles, word games, memory boosters, reading exercises, healthy choices for healthy living, and more.

This activity book will bring happiness and satisfaction to those who enjoy puzzles, playing word games, or solving math problems. We understand this demographic may require additional time or guidance, so we designed the content with these individuals in mind. Our goal is to ensure that we are making the puzzles simple and fun - but still providing an engaging experience no matter your reading skill or comprehension level.

Whether they are differently abled or simply a lover of puzzles, our workbook is perfect for spending time with your loved ones, helping to improve their mood, vocabulary, and overall life satisfaction.

Dear Reader,

If you enjoy puzzles, games with words, or doing math - we have a good book for you! We think you will enjoy our puzzle book!

Finish word searches, math problems, spelling tests, and read short stories! Take your pick from puzzles, memory games, learning healthy habits, and much more.

They are all here in this workbook for you to enjoy!

We have designed this book for you to do independently with little help! You can go in order or skip to the pages you like best.

We hope you have fun and enjoy your time using this activity book.

chapter one

Memory Boosters, Reminiscent
Reminders and Music

```
P L F N H
B A I W A
J U S K P
O G I T P
Y H I T Y
```

FIND THESE WORDS

1. JOY
2. LAUGH
3. PAST
4. HAPPY

Name 3 things that make you happy

_____

_____

_____

seek joy

Can you recall...?

Read this short story with your loved one, and guide them to rewrite it on the following page.

Martha wanted a pet to keep her company. She thinks a cat would be a good companion.

Martha decided to go to the nearest adoption center and view the kittens.

Martha found a black and white kitten to adopt and she named her 'Mittens'.

Martha brought Mittens home about six months ago, and she is a great cuddler.

Can you recall...?

Guide your loved one to rewrite it on this page.

Martha wanted a _____ to keep her company. She thinks a _____ would be a good companion.

Martha decided to go to the nearest adoption center and view the _____.

Martha found a _____ and _____ kitten to adopt and she named her 'Mittens'.

Martha brought Mittens home about _____ months ago, and she is a great cuddler.

Tell me more...

What did you want to be when you grew up?

_____

Do you have a favorite place in the world?

_____

What were you scared of as a kid?

_____

Do you or have you had any pets?

_____

Talking with your loved one about their past will help them focus on remembering important information. Still, it can help them identify moments of joy they have had. The key to improving their mood is to maintain a healthy level of pleasant reminiscing and communication to foster a connection through the past you've experienced together.

Where are we going next?

John needs to pay his bills at the local bank. He needs $200 in cash to bring to the bank teller.

He needs to be there by 5:00 p.m. before it closes. It is currently 3:00 p.m. It takes 10 minutes to reach the bank.

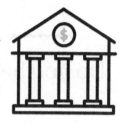

After paying his bills, he will buy dinner and go home.
Where is John going?

_____

How much money does he need to bring?

_____

If he wants to arrive on time, when should he leave?

_____

Where is he expected to go after buying dinner?

_____

Let's match these objects!

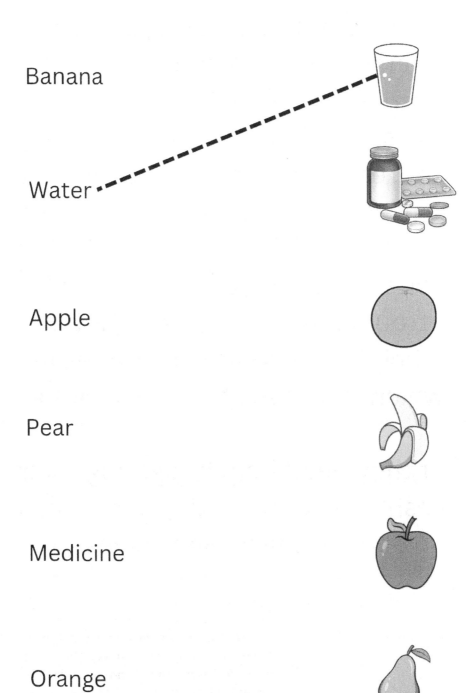

Banana

Water

Apple

Pear

Medicine

Orange

One of the challenges with dementia is remembering to do important tasks. One of the best ways to help them remember is to refresh them on the information necessary to complete the tasks.

For example, if your loved one has trouble remembering their bills, help them create envelopes in which they can store their money.

If they need help budgeting their cash - be gentle and guide them in counting it themselves.

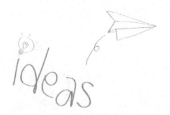

Another helpful step is to guide them to break the process down further. If they have a $25 cell phone bill, $25 electric bill, and $25 water bill, do not put it in one envelope as $75. Instead, use paperclips and Post-its to identify the cash groups.

If your loved one has appointments and medical issues, one thing you can do to help them remember important dates is to help them write these dates down themselves.

A daily calendar is an excellent way to help them remember important dates as they come. This differs from a weekly planner - every day will be presented as an entirely new page.

The next page is a probable example of a daily task planner for your loved one.

Today we must:

1 _____

2 _____

3 _____

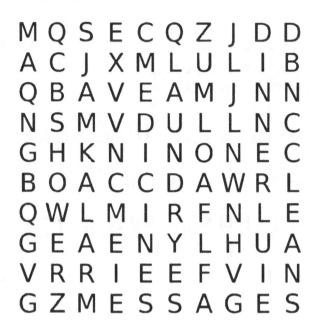

```
M Q S E C Q Z J D D
A C J X M L U L I B
Q B A V E A M J N N
N S M V D U L L N C
G H K N I N O N E C
B O A C C D A W R L
Q W L M I R F N L E
G E A E N Y L H U A
V R R I E E F V I N
G Z M E S S A G E S
```

1. Medicine
2. Dinner
3. Clean
4. Messages
5. Laundry
6. Shower
7. Alarm

Using words and reading words like these frequently can help the brain make them a more permanent thought. You want to help your loved one remind themselves to do these things because it helps them remember more in the long run.

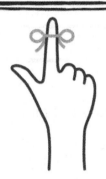

"HOW TO WRITE A TO-DO LIST"

TO DO LIST

1. GET YOUR PAPER AND PEN
2. WRITE 3 IMPORTANT THINGS TO DO TODAY
3. POST IT ON YOUR REFRIGERATOR
4. CHECK OFF WHEN YOU FINISH A TASK

What three things do you need to do tomorrow?

1. _____
2. _____
3. _____

YOU'VE GOT THIS!

chapter two

Sensory Activities for Everyone

Do you smell that?

Scent is a very, very powerful tool in triggering memories. Have you ever been sitting somewhere and smelled something familiar and all of a sudden there are feelings being stirred in you? That's because the brain connects memories to scents deeply. You can use scents to help ignite memories and feelings in your loved ones! Below are some examples of scents that may evoke a powerful feeling or fond memory.

Christmas
Candy Canes
Cinnamon
Turkey Dinner

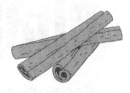

Autumn
Nutmeg
Pumpkin Pie
Spiced Apple

Vacations
Cut Grass
Sea Breeze
Sunscreen

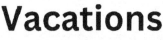

Childhood
Birthday Cake
Favorite Meals
Mom's Perfume

Please consult a health care professional before using essential oils for aromatherapy. There are dangers to overusing scents, for example excessive amounts of peppermint can impair breathing. Please do not start using aromatherapy until you have a comprehensive understanding of your loved ones needs, allergies and state of health.

What does this remind you of?

You need essential oils as follows:
- Peppermint
- Cinnamon
- Coconut
- Basil

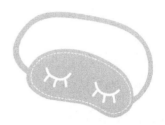

Have your loved one close their eyes, and let them smell one of the scents.

Ask them if they enjoy it, what it reminds them of, such as food or holidays, and if it brings back any memories.

Which smell is your favorite?

Scavenger Hunt!

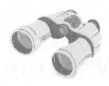

Walk around your home
and see if you can find the
following of items!

Perfume

A Set of Keys

A Left Sock

Sunglasses

Go for a walk with your
loved one and see if
you can find things
like this outside!

A White Car

A Song Bird

A Traffic Light

A Dog on a Walk

You can incorporate sensory activities in your everyday activities.

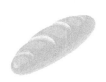 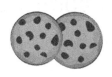 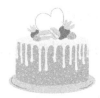

Sensory activities are good ways to enjoy time together and create something fun! For example, making dough. You can use dough for a multitude of baked goods, combining ingredients and kneading it are great ways to experience different smells, tastes, and feelings.

Three Ingredient Dough

1/2 cup whole-wheat flour

1/2 cup fat-free plain Greek yogurt

3/4 tsp. baking powder

Can be used as pizza dough or bread. Bake between 350-400° for 5-15 minutes to your individual tastes. Add a pinch of salt if you'd like.

Cozy Corner

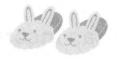

Gather some of comfort items. Some examples include:

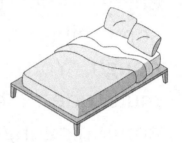

- Pillow
- Blanket
- Stuffed Animal
- Favorite Book
- Photo Album
- Comfy Clothes

Sit together every once in awhile and get comfy! Find the softest clothes and blankets, turn on a movie or read a book together. Being close and in a comfortable environment will help promote relaxation, touch on sensory needs, and foster and closer bond over you time spent together reminiscing.

```
S T S Z M F P U P P
B Y H L W S C I V M
P E C M U R L D F W
W I D O D C E B D W
T W D T M L N S C A
P G H Q I F I H T S
U R Y F I M Y V G H
R M B J U Z E M J L
B F V V T K F V K J
N H X C Y A K O B E
```

1. Bedtime
2. Comfy
3. Rest
4. Wash

Tic Tac Toe

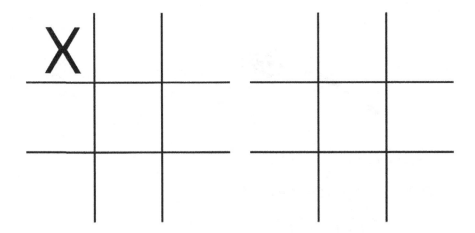

Photo Prompts

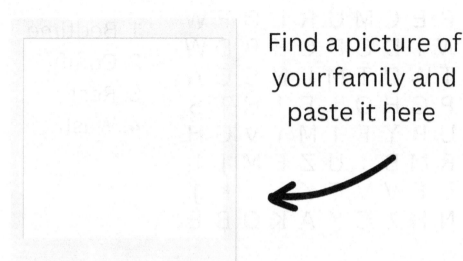

Find a picture of your family and paste it here

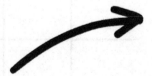

Add a picture of your favorite place in this frame

Add your 3 favorite pictures!

Maybe a picture of your pet? What's your favorite memory? Do you have a picture of a loved one?

Autumn Leaves is an easy memory and matching game for seniors that encourages them outside to breathe in the fresh air, stretch their legs and change their environment.

To play, follow these steps:

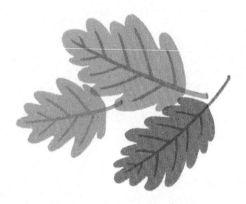

- Pick up various leaves, focusing on different colours and shapes.
- Head back inside.
- Support your loved one in trying to remember the name of the leaf and who picked it.

Music is amazing

Music can stimulate the brain to recall memories, words, tunes, skills and much more. Some of the best ways to bring joy to someone is to play their favorite song. Ask your loved ones what their favorite songs are, maybe make them a playlist or turn on some music together when you do day to day tasks like housework or cooking meals. You may catch them singing along flawlessly!

What type of music do you like?

_____

What's your favorite song?

_____

Can you play any instruments?

_____

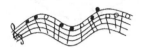

Let's Sing!

We are the champions,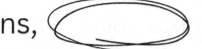

We'll keep on fighting till the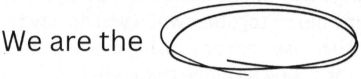

We are the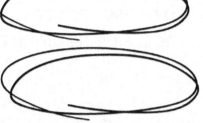

We are the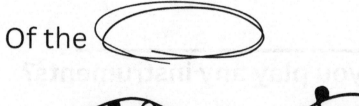

No time for losers

'Cause we are the champions

Of the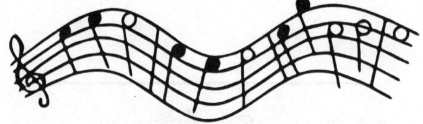

Let's sing!

Never gonna give you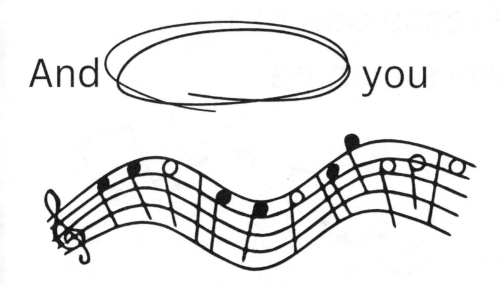

Never gonna let you

Never gonna run around

And   you

Let's SING!

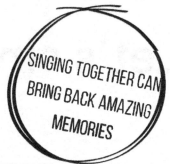

SINGING TOGETHER CAN BRING BACK AMAZING MEMORIES

You are my sunshine,
My only
You make me happ
When skies are
You'll never know dear
How much I   you
Please don't take
My sunshine

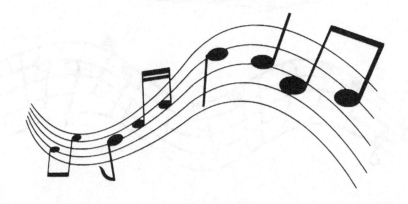

chapter three

Artistic Expression - Let's get creative!

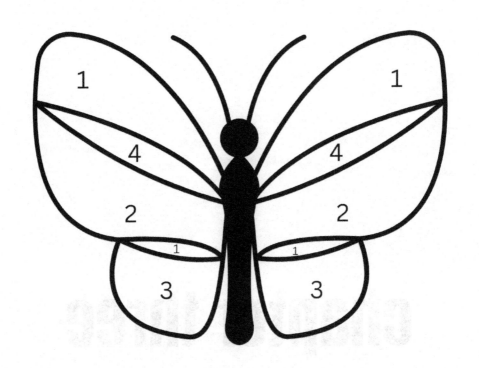

1 - Pink   3 - Purple
2 - Blue   4 - Yellow

**Try coloring this butterfly
according to the color legend!**

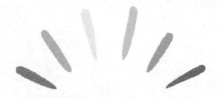

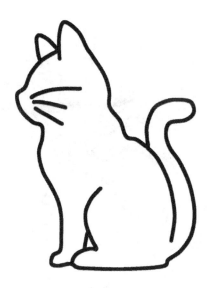

Color this cat brown.

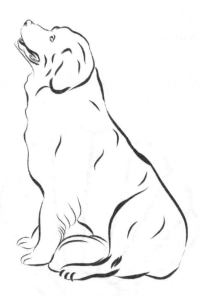

Color this dog yellow

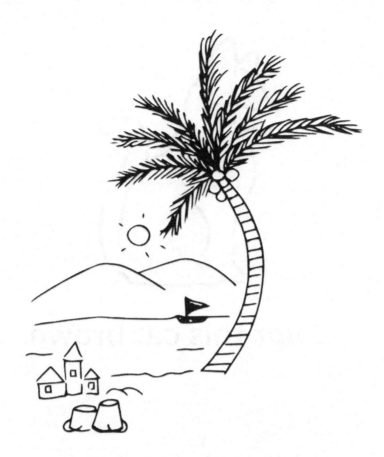

Color the beach scene

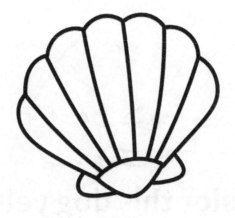

Color the seashell

Color these delicious foods!

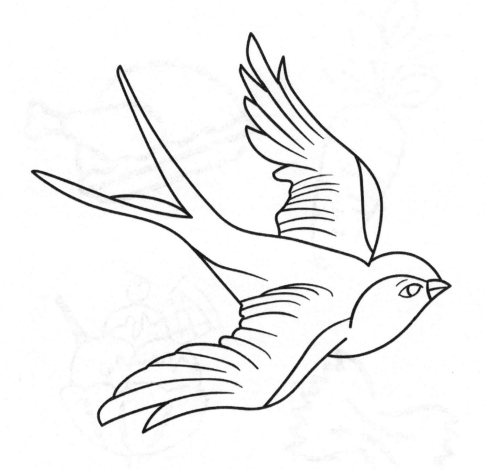

Color this beautiful sparrow!

You can find sparrows and other
small birds outside in every city
and town around the world. Go for
a walk and see how many different
kinds you can spot!

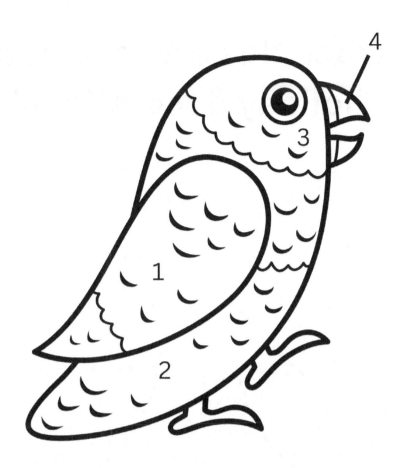

1 - Pink   3 - Purple
2 - Blue   4 - Yellow

Trace this tree and add holiday decorations!

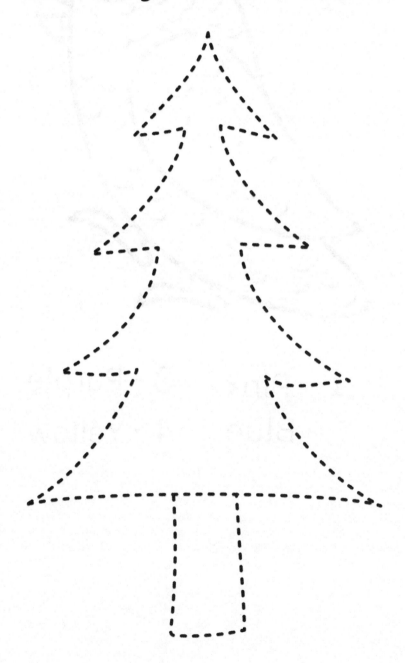

Trace these birds and add some color!

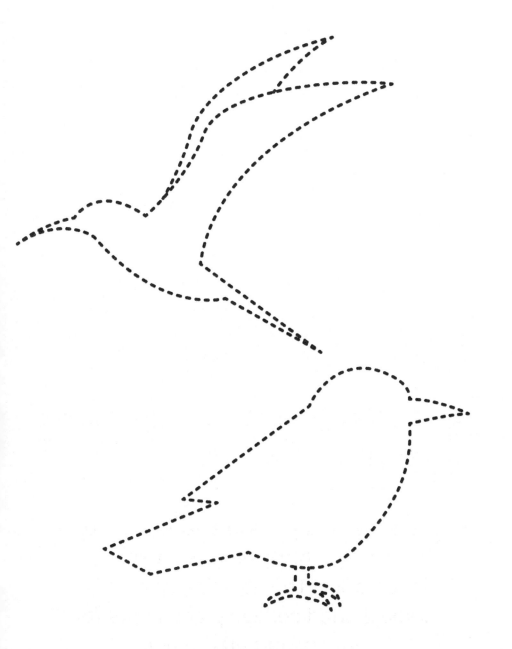

Make a little collage of your favorite things!

Making collages are a good way to help trigger old memories with your loved ones. The next few pages are some guided collage placements for you! Try and fill them up!

Make a little collage of your favorite places!

You can draw or find photos in pictures or magazines to make your collages!

Make a little collage of your favorite animals!

You can draw or find photos in pictures or magazines to make your collages!

chapter four

Brain teasers - Games, Crosswords,
Wordsearch and more!

There have been many amazing research studies in recent years that state that the effectiveness of "brain games" for helping those who are living with cognitive disabilities, such as dementia. There are many stimulating and fun brain games for dementia patients that caregivers and their loved ones can utilize.

Games can offer both social and mental stimulation which is excellent for promoting memories, while "exercising" the brain.

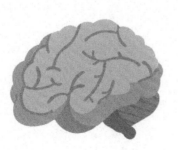

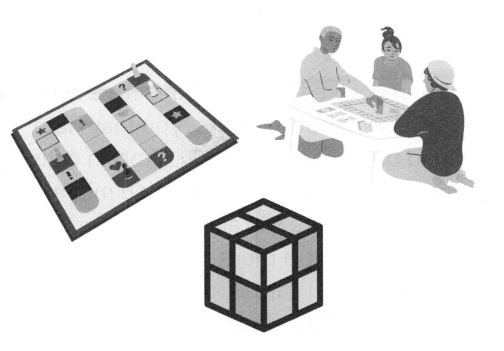

Games that include matching pictures of people, objects or animals with their corresponding name gives memory care participants a visual component to connect to a word. This is especially recommended for flash cards that might include family members, everyday items or exotic animals

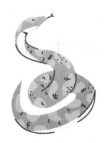
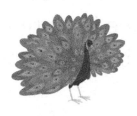
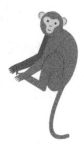

When you keep your brain active with exercises or other tasks, you may help build up a reserve supply of brain cells and links between them. You might even grow new brain cells. Experts think the extra mental activity from stimuli Fromm games, puzzles and tasks may protect the brain by strengthening connections between its cells.

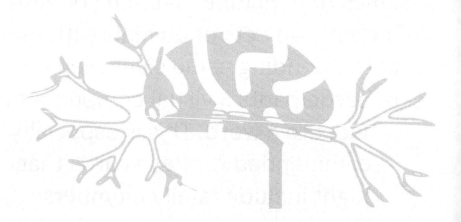

Check online for new games and apps every once in awhile - research is always bringing us new things!

Crossword Puzzle!

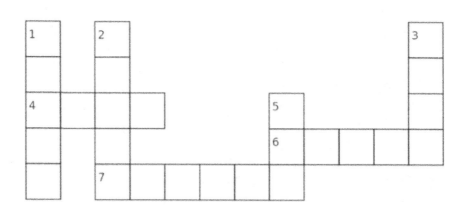

Down

1

2

3

5

Across

4

6

7

Water Tree
Bread Apple
Home Dinner
Car

```
X H K H O L I D A Y
R Q J C D D Z O X E
Z P E L S J O F F I
V A C A T I O N R G
F K T F R I Z J I A
X A Z U L Q T F E M
U K M N A I V G N E
B H K I C E Z V D S
Y G A C L Y F H S C
X W F Q H Y U G N H
```

1. Holiday
2. Family
3. Friends
4. Fun
5. Vacation
6. Games

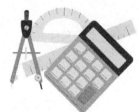

Can you solve these math problems?

	+		+	6	11
+	■	+	■	+	
	+		+		15
+	■	+	■	+	
7	+		+		19
16		9		20	

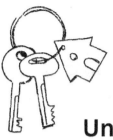

Unscramble these words!

YSEK   _____

OMHE   _____

BKAN   _____

ONMYE   _____

USB   _____

IETM   _____

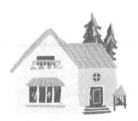

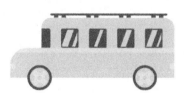

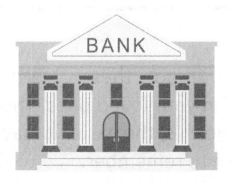

Let's Have a Spelling Bee

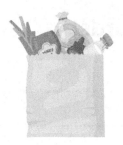

_____

_____

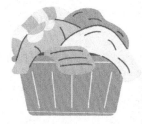

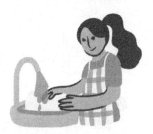

_____

_____

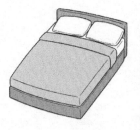

Spell and read these words outloud with your loved ones. The more you do this, the easier it may be for them to remember.

Shopping
Laundry
Cleaning
Bedtime

```
F Q L N A C R S W Y
H R L E D G Y O G A
P E U R J F D Z Y W
Y P A I R P T I Q U
N Y H L T V K V X R
K D I E T E K I M W
B E R S W H J B Z A
V C D P V Y Y Q O T
D R O K L B F H Z E
U X S Q Z P V O H R
```

1. Yoga
2. Water
3. Healthy
4. Diet
5. Fruit

Circle your favorite fruit

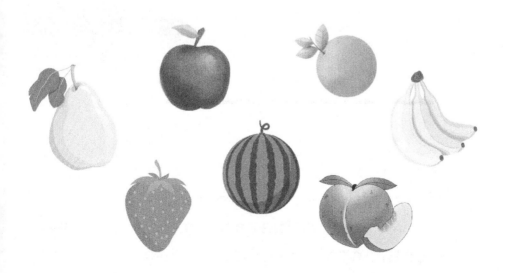

Let's Have a Spelling Bee 🐝

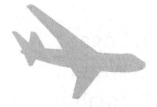

_____

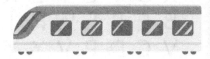

_____

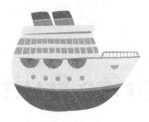

_____

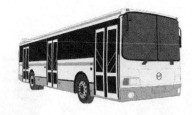

_____

Spell and read these words outloud with your loved ones. The more you do this, the easier it may be for them to remember.

Plane
Train
Boat
Bus

Can you match these?

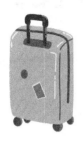

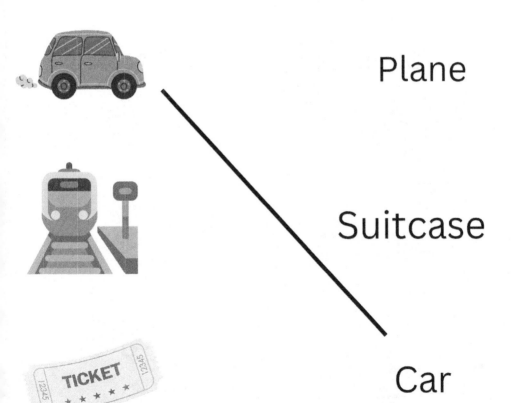

Ticket

Train

Plane

Suitcase

Car

Crossword Puzzle!

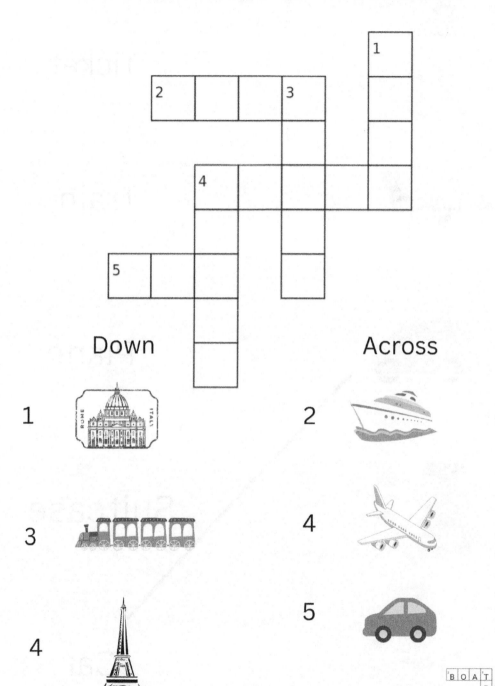

Down

1

3

4

Across

2

4

5

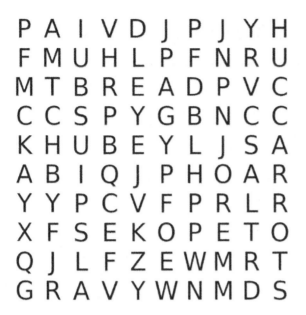

```
P A I V D J P J Y H
F M U H L P F N R U
M T B R E A D P V C
C C S P Y G B N C C
K H U B E Y L J S A
A B I Q J P H O A R
Y Y P C V F P R L R
X F S E K O P E T O
Q J L F Z E W M R T
G R A V Y W N M D S
```

1. Pepper
2. Salt
3. Bread
4. Chicken
5. Carrots
6. Gravy

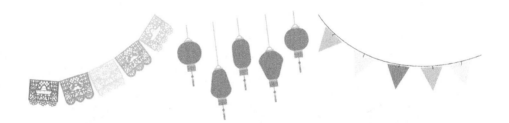

What ethnic foods are your favorite?

_____

_____

_____

Unscramble these words

OCOIEK   _____

BRDEA   _____

EPLPA   _____

GREAON   _____

EJUCI   _____

TAWRE   _____

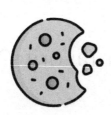 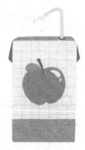 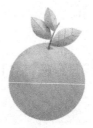

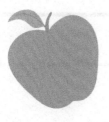 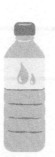 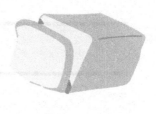

Let's Have a Spelling 🐝

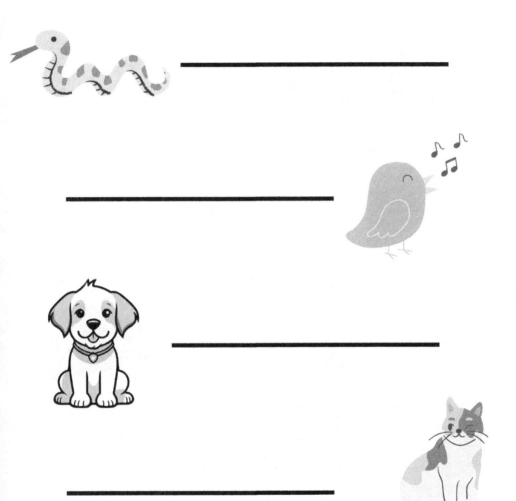

_____

_____

_____

_____

Spell and read these words outloud with your loved ones. The more you do this, the easier it may be for them to remember.

Snake
Bird
Dog
Cat

Try to write equations that equal five!

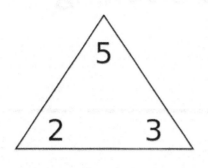

____ + ____ = ____

____ + ____ = ____

____ − ____ = ____

____ − ____ = ____

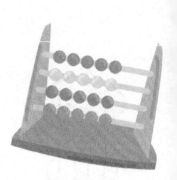

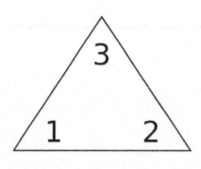

____ + ____ = ____

____ + ____ = ____

____ − ____ = ____

____ − ____ = ____

Patterns

Follow along and complete the rest of the pattern!

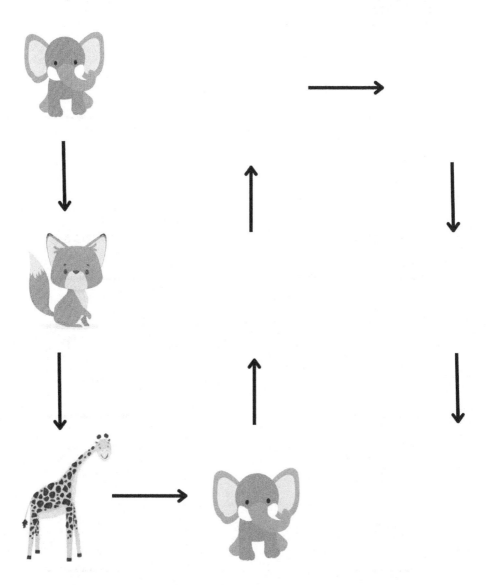

SAFARI SCRAMBLE!

- Unscramble the letters to name the animals! -

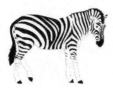

EZRBA

_____

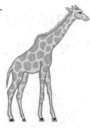

FAFEIRG

_____

ONYKEM

_____

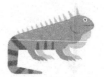

GIUNAA

_____

AKSNE

_____

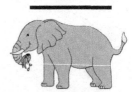

NEHPATEL

_____

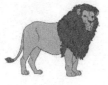

INLO

_____

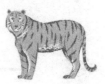

RGTEI

_____

Super Word Search

```
L Y J P P Q X U Y T
L T M X U B F P Z D
H B B A I Z Q M V G
Z M S G T E Z I Q I
T A T C A C C L E K
F T R C A M H U E V
N H I L B R E I H S
M Y C V E G D S N X
Q L K Q M X S S E G
M U S G Q X I B U B
```

1. Puzzles
2. Cards
3. Matching
4. Tricks
5. Math
6. Games

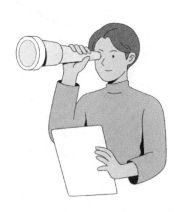

Match the animal to it's product!

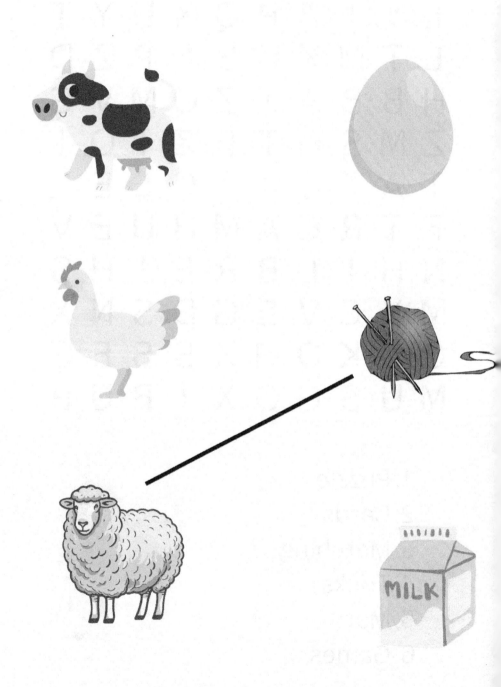

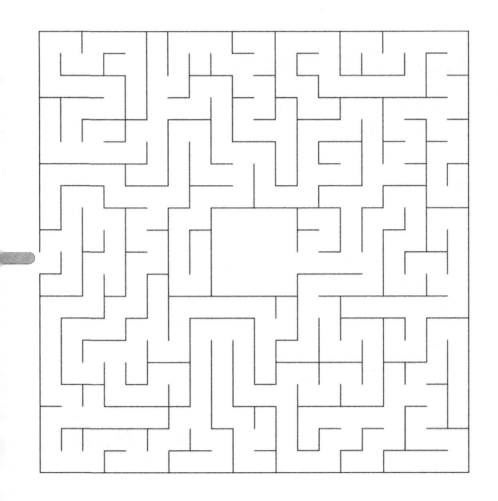

Can you find your way out of the center?

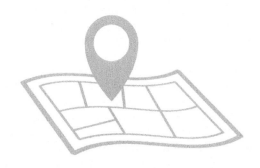

Word Scrambles

Unscramble the animals, then match their name to their picture

1. HNETLPAE _____
2. HIFS _____
3. GTIRE _____
4. IADRLZ _____
5. MTRSEHA _____

chapter five

Healthy Movement - Yoga, Stretching, Dancing!

Let's Have a Spelling Bee

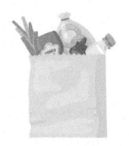
_____

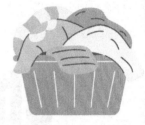
_____

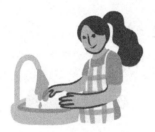
_____

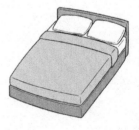
_____

Spell and read these words outloud with your loved ones. The more you do this, the easier it may be for them to remember.

Shopping
Laundry
Cleaning
Bedtime

Get moving!

Exercise is important to everyone, and working out or doing yoga a few times a week can drastically improve the quality of people's lives.

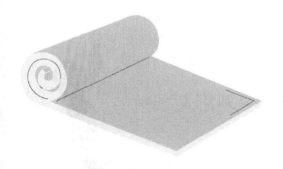

Research shows that just ten minutes a day can help release hormones that will help improve your overall mood, and health at the same time. You can increase your energy levels, stamina and reduce anxiety if you implement an exercise routine.

Some great types of low impact exercise include:

- **Yoga**
- **Brisk Walking**
- **Strength Training**
- **Swimming**

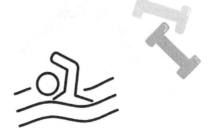

Gentle Yoga Poses

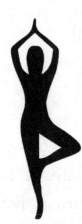

- Stand on one leg
- Rest your foot on your knees
- Raise your hands above your head
- Hold for 20 seconds and repeat

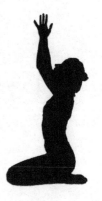

- Kneel on the floor
- Raise your arms above your head
- Take deep breath
- Repeat

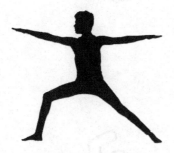

- Feet Apart
- Turn your body
- Raise your arms
- Deep breathes
- Repeat

Online Exercise Programs!

Brain Gym - YouTube

https://youtu.be/DJt6ORwxKmE

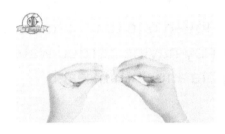

Simple hand tricks
and counting games!

Yoga with Kassandra - YouTube

https://youtu.be/EvMTrP8eRvM

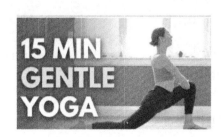

Low impact yoga
exercises for all
strength levels

Stay Healthy!

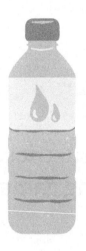

Did you drink water today?

Hydration is key to a healthy happy body, especially when exercising.. Help remind your loved one to remember to drink water by having bottled water available and within reach.

Make Good Choices

Helped your loved one maintain a healthy diet by having fresh fruits and vegetables on hand and easily accessible. They will help with hydration, fibre, and vitamin intake. If your loved one is diabetic, opt for high fibre vegetables instead of fruits.

```
F Q L N A C R S W Y
H R L E D G Y O G A
P E U R J F D Z Y W
Y P A I R P T I Q U
N Y H L T V K V X R
K D I E T E K I M W
B E R S W H J B Z A
V C D P V Y Y Q O T
D R O K L B F H Z E
U X S Q Z P V O H R
```

1. Yoga
2. Water
3. Healthy
4. Diet
5. Fruit

Circle your favorite fruit

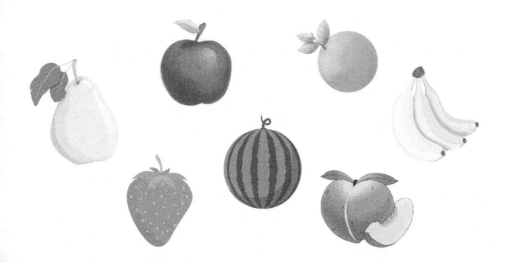

Crossword Puzzle!

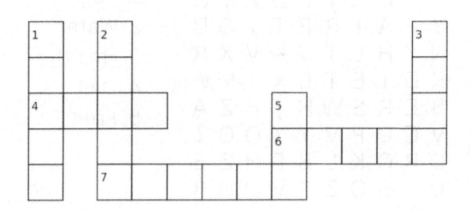

Down

1

2

3

5

Across

4

6

7

Water	Tree
Bread	Apple
Home	Dinner
Car	

Name your favorite things!
Write or draw them below!

What is your favorite food?

What is your favorite sport?

What is your favorite ice cream flavor?

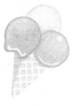

May I have this dance?

We have explained how music can help boost mood and memory, but did you know dance can also help with that? If your loved one has a favorite song, try and put it on. Ask them how they feel, ask if they would like to dance with you!

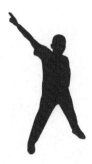

Depending on where you are located, you may be able to find locations near you who actually host community dances! A good way to find out is to use Google and search 'community dance events' near me and see if there are any that are inclusive for people with disabilities!

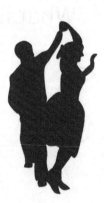

There's a possibility to have lots of fun and make new friends in the process.

Calm Breathing

Square Breathing:
- Breathe in through your nose for 4 seconds
- Hold for 4 seconds
- Breathe out for 4 seconds
- Hold for 4 seconds
- Repeat these steps while tracing a small square with your finger on the table

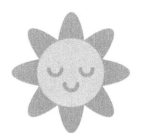

Take 5 Breathing:
- Spread your hand open and stretch your fingers
- Take a deep breathe while you trace one finger up, and down
- Repeat the breathes until you've traced all 5 fingers

Belly Breathing:
- Place one hand on your stomach
- Breathe in slow while imagining an inflating balloon in your stomach
- Exhale slowly, declaring the balloon
- Repeat three times

Brain Training

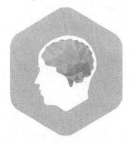

Elevate - Brain Training: Trains with memory games, math questions, and word games!

Happify: For Stress and Worry: Helps emotional regulation with meditation, activities, and games.

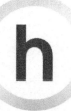

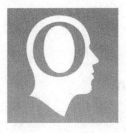

CogniFit - Brain Training: Improves your memory, concentration, coordination, and more with games dedicated to each concept.

chapter six

Armchair travel! View the
world at home!

Where in the world .. ?

Have you travelled before? Some of the best memories come from travelling. If you haven't travelled that's okay, because in the era we live in today we can experience the beauty of other countries thanks to the internet!

Can you name these monuments?

_____

_____

Let's Have a Spelling Bee

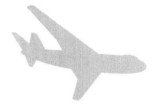

_____

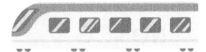

_____

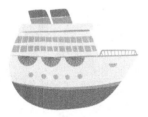

_____

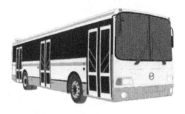

_____

Spell and read these words outloud with your loved ones. The more you do this, the easier it may be for them to remember.

Plane
Train
Boat
Bus

Unscramble these cities!

SARPI   _____

EMRO   _____

ETNHAS   _____

LNDNOO   _____

OORNOTT   _____

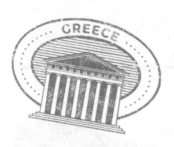

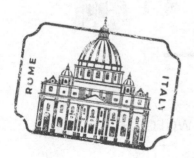

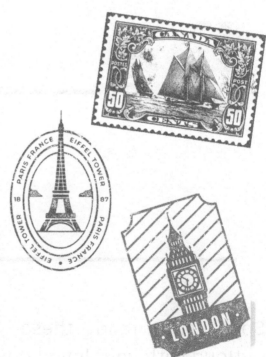

Paris
Rome
Athens
London
Toronto

Let's plan a trip!

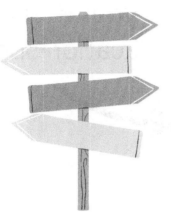

To go on your trip to your friend's city for a visit, you will need $70 for your train ticket. You need to pack a suitcase with days worth of clothes. You also need to remember your sunscreen!

How long will you be staying?

_____

How much is your train ticket?

_____

It's important to remember your :

_____

Travel Memory Prompts

Paste a picture of your dream vacation spot.

Paste a picture of your favorite travel memory.

Can you match these?

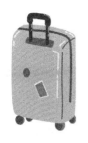

Ticket

Train

Plane

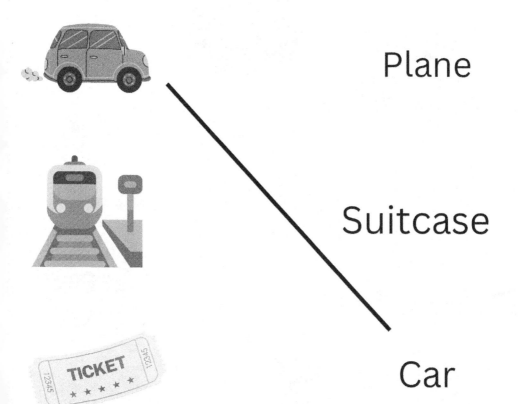

Suitcase

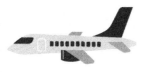

Car

If you were invited to go camping for the weekend, what are the things that you need to bring?

Circle them below!

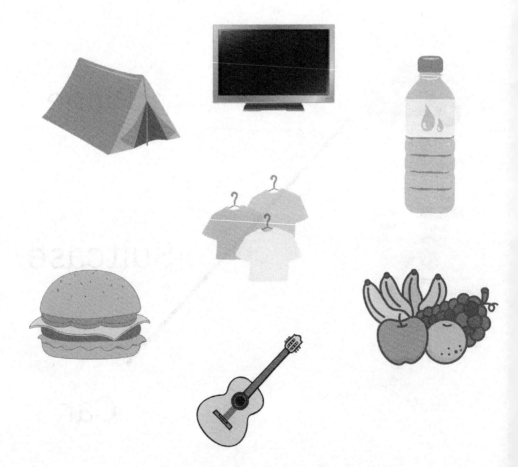

Travel at Home!

There are apps you can use with your phone or Virtual Reality headsets that will allow you to explore and experience travel from the comfort of your own home! Helped your loved one download and configure the apps so they can enjoy the beauty of the world from their favorite chair!

- Google Earth VR
- Everest VR
- theBlu
- National Geographic VR

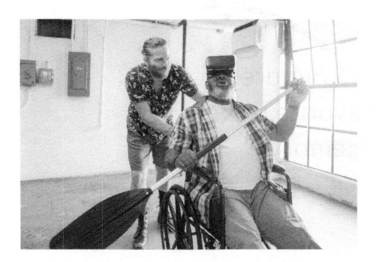

Travel Memory Prompts

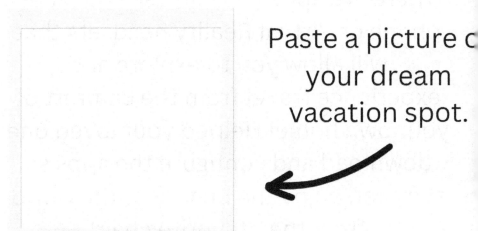

Paste a picture of your dream vacation spot.

Paste a picture of your favorite travel memory.

Photo Prompts

Find a picture of
your family and
paste it here

Add a picture of
your favorite place
in this frame

chapter seven

Culinary Adventures - Let's
cook! Let's Eat!

A healthy diet is of course important for overall health, but it may be even more beneficial for preventing and slowing the progression of cognitive diseases, and help with mental function. Diet is not the only factor in prevention, however. There are many other things to consider, such as genes, stress levels, and mental stimulation - but brain food while maintaining a good sleep schedule, managing your stress and incorporating mental stimulation such as solving puzzles or hobbies can all help maintain good mental fitness. Eating "brain food" might help with your memory!

- Berries
- Fish
- Nuts and Seeds
- Leafy Greens
- Lean Meat
- Avocados
- Tomatoes

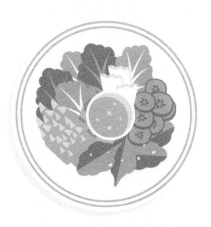

Super Smoothie

Help your loved one make a 'super smoothie', packed full of nutrients that are great for your brain!

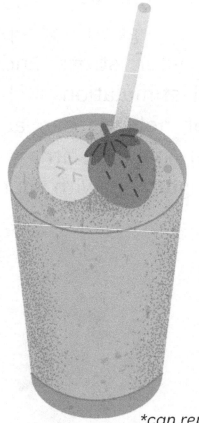

Blueberries
Strawberries
Kale & Spinach
Hemp Seeds
Greek Yogurt*
Coconut Milk

Blend with ice
and enjoy!

*can replace yogurt with kefir or
dairy substitute*

Do you have a favorite recipe?

Sit with your loved one and reminisce about some of the lovely meals they've had in their lives, maybe on vacation in their favorite country or on holidays with family. Ask them which were there favorites and see if they can write a short recipe below!

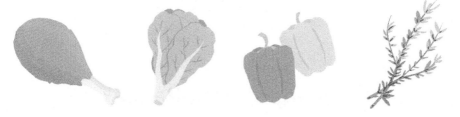

What vegetables do we need?

What type of protein do we need?

What type of herbs do we need?

Let's Eat!

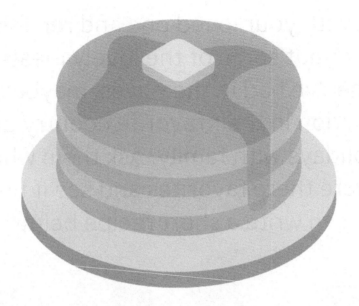

Three Ingredient Pancakes

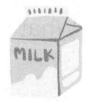

2 Bananas
1/2 Cup Flour
1/2 cup milk

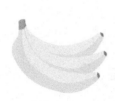

- Smash your bananas into a paste
- Add milk, and slowly sift in flour until combined.
- Drop by the spoonful on the skillet
- Flip when you see the tiny bubbles popping!

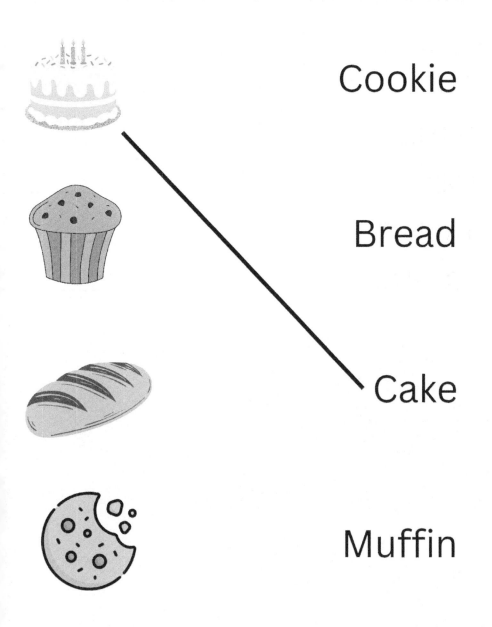

Cookie

Bread

Cake

Muffin

Have you baked any of these before?

Unscramble these baking words!

GGE   _____

ORFLU   _____

LMIK   _____

TRUEBT   _____

ERCMA   _____

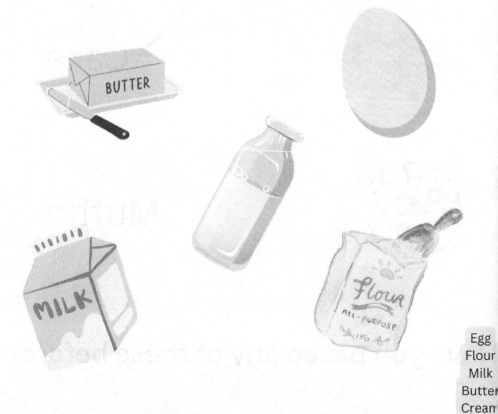

Egg
Flour
Milk
Butter
Cream

Peanut Butter Banana Oat Bars

----

1. **3 Ripe Bananas**
2. **2 Cups Dry Oats**
3. **6tbsp Peanut Butter**

**Preheat the oven to 350 degrees.
Mix all your ingredients in a bowl
and press firmly into a dish.
Set a timer and bake for 18-20
minutes.**

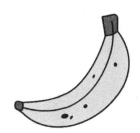

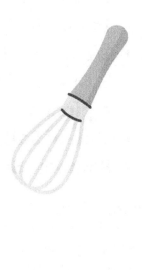

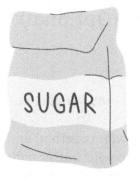

Funfetti Birthday Cake!

INGREDIENTS

- 4 and 1/2 tbsp of Butter
- 1/2 Cup of White Sugar
- 1tsp of Vanilla
- 1 and 1/2 Eggs
- 1/2 Cup of Milk
- 1 Cup of Flour
- A pinch of Salt
- 1tsp of Salt
- Rainbow Sprinkles (Optional)

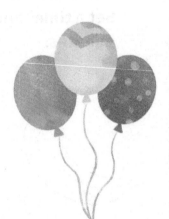

INSTRUCTIONS

1. Pregeat oven to 350 degrees
2. Mix together the butter, sugar, and vanilla until fluffy
3. Add in your eggs
4. Sift your flour and baking powder together, and alternate adding the milk and the flour mixture into your butter and eggs
5. Place in a cake pan and bake for 20-25 minutes

Food Around the World

Think of a meal from your country, and list some of the ingredients you need to make it.

Your Meal: _____

Ingredients

1. _____
2. _____
3. _____
4. _____
5. _____

Your Rainbow Diet

Pick the foods and sort them by their colour in the rainbow! Write it's name in the arch, and colour it in!

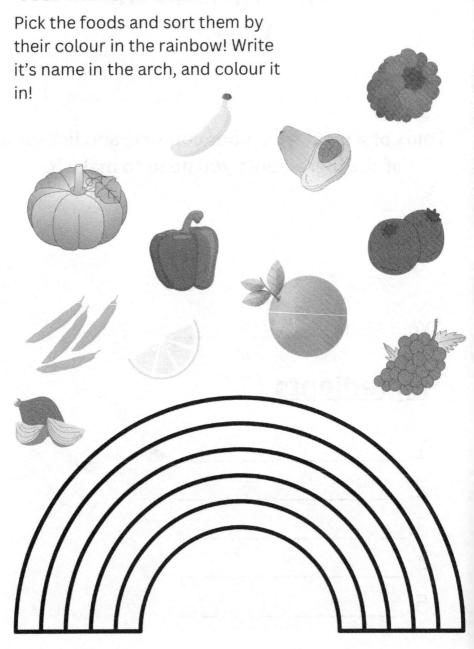

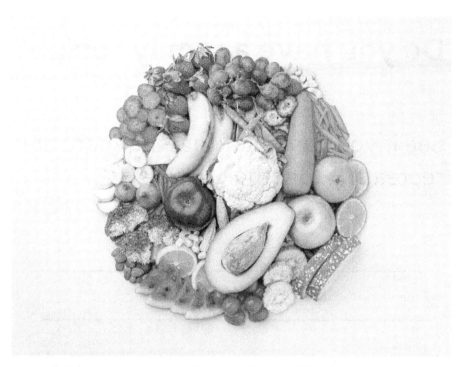

- See how many of these Fruits and Vegetables you can name! -

------------------   ------------------   ------------------

------------------   ------------------   ------------------

------------------   ------------------   ------------------

------------------   ------------------   ------------------

------------------   ------------------   ------------------

------------------   ------------------   ------------------

Do you have a family recipe?

See if you can put it together here and recreate it together!

_____

_____

_____

_____

_____

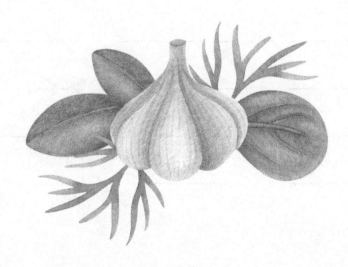

chapter eight

Animal Therapy! Pets are
amazing!

Do you have a pet?

Animals enhance human well-being in many ways, from providing companionship to improving mental health to instilling empathy and support in others lives.

Their presence can help lessen the effects of dementia such as anxiety, restlessness, irritability, depression and loneliness. By being friendly and nonthreatening, pets can help people with dementia interact more, which is sometimes not possible in social situations with other adults.

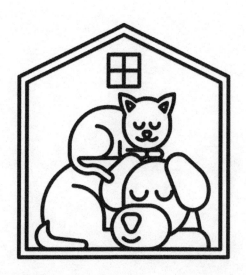

If keeping a pet for yourself or your loved one isn't something you are able to accommodate, try finding some of your favorite animals outside. Birds are great for watching, and they actually recognize you if you see them frequently.

Try buying a small bag of wild bird seed and go outside. You'll begin to develop a routine with the neighborhood birds in no time!

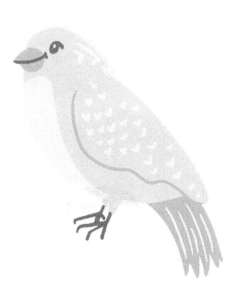

The Joy for All Pet Companions are excellent robotic plush animal cats, kittens, and puppies.
Because they run on batteries, they can move, respond realistically to being touched or cuddled, and purr, meow, and bark.

This is one of multiple companies who provide robotic style companions for people with cognitive disabilities.

Some companies include:

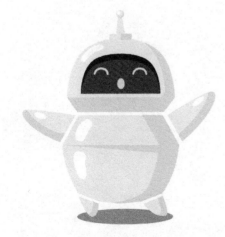

- Ageless Innovations
- Bittle Robotic
- Anko
- Dogness iPet

Many people with dementia benefit from comforting dolls or teddies, or interacting with lifelike robotic animals.

Some studies have shown that a 'fake' pet can bring many of the same calming effects as a real pet, so this might be a good option to explore first.

There are some apps below you can use with your loved one to simulate caring for a real pet any time of the day!

My Tamagotchi Forever
BANDAI NAMCO Entertainment Europe
Contains ads • In-app purchases

Old Friends Dog Game
Runaway
Contains ads • In-app purchases

with My CAT
neilo
Contains ads • In-app purchases

Pet Pals
PlayPals Games
Contains ads • In-app purchases

Memory Matching

Draw lines to connect the animals to the correct match

A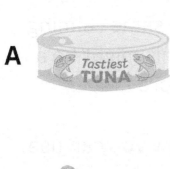

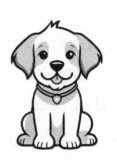 **1**

B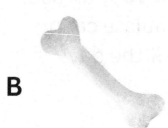

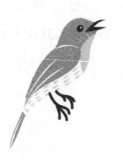 **2**

C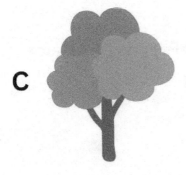

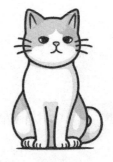 **3**

Animal Search

Circle the animas off of the list:

- **Cat**
- **Bird**
- **Elephant**
- **Racoon**
- **Dog**

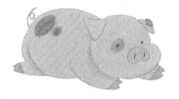
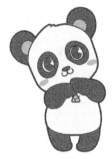
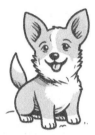
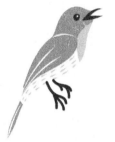
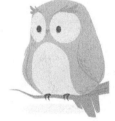
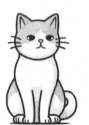
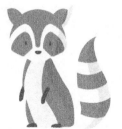
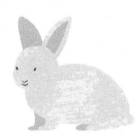

Take your dog for a walk!

Complete the maze through the grass to find your way to the dog park

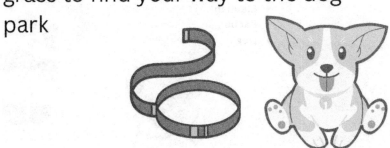

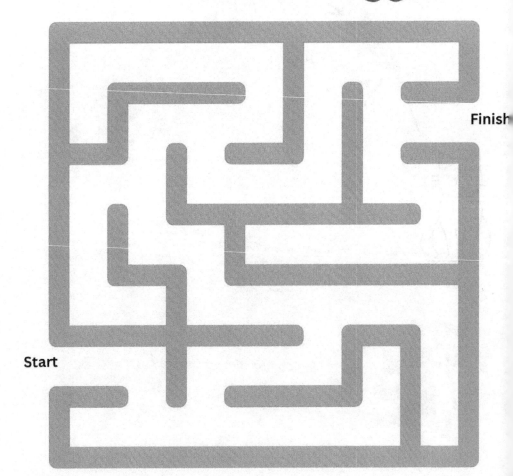

Finish

Start

You have a new puppy! Use the list and circle what items you will need

- Name Tag and Collar
- Food Dish
- Dog House
- Toy Bone
- Dog Brush

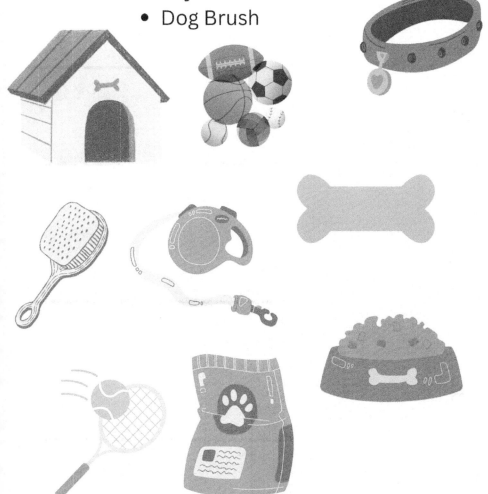

Grooming your pets is an important part of being their owner. What do you need to give the dog a bath?

1. _____

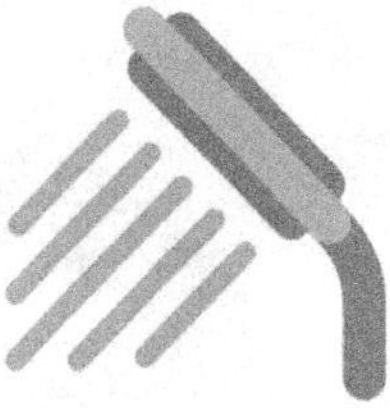

2. _____

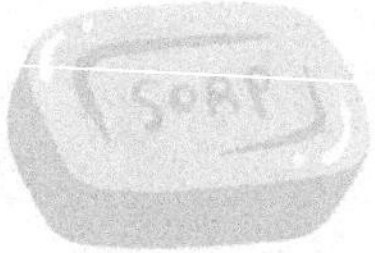

3. _____

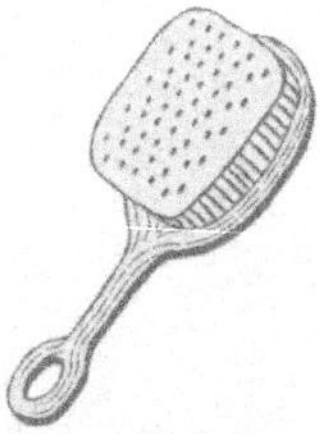

4. _____

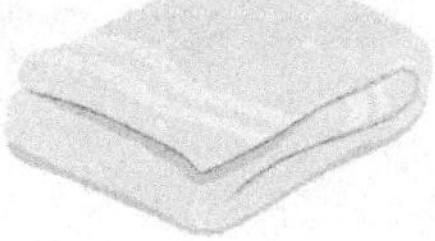

Having a pet can help improve many areas of life in a Dementia Patient:

- Can improve their independence
- Helps improve their confidence and self-esteem
- Can help them with understanding and connecting

Connect the dots to complete the pets.

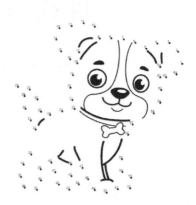

_____

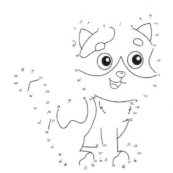

_____

chapter nine

Mindfulness - Relaxing is important for your health!

Have you tried meditation?

There are many research studies that show that meditation can help relax and ease tension for everyone! It's a centuries-old method of clearing your mind and enabling yourself to completely relax. Sometimes it is hard to get the hang of, but even trying is a great step!

Give it a shot!

1. Sit somewhere comfortable
2. Close your eyes
3. Try to focus on something peaceful
4. Try and attempt to stop thinking about your worries and stressors for just awhile!

- Let your breath flow as deep down into your belly as is comfortable, without forcing it.
- Try breathing in through your nose and out through your mouth.
- Breathe in gently and regularly. Some people find it helpful to count steadily from 1 to 5. You may not be able to reach 5 at first.
- Then let it flow out gently, counting from 1 to 5 again, if you find this helpful.
- Keep doing this for at least 5 minutes

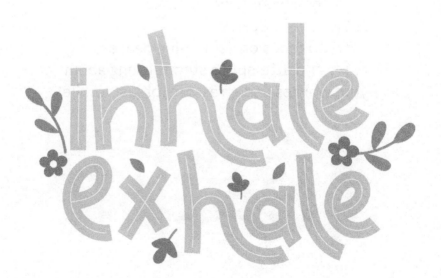

YOGA

Slower practices like Hatha yoga or Kundalini yoga often involves meditation and chanting during the class, ideal for tapping into your "inner peace". Finding a local class is a good way to connect with others in your community as well!

YouTube also has a plethora of videos available that can also help you practice various forms of yoga!

Virtual Care Taking

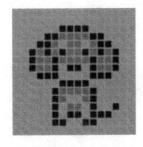

Dogotchi: Take care of your virtual tomagatchi pet!

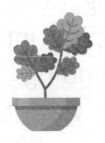

Terrarium Garden Idle: Water, Feed, and Grow your plants to level up your terrarium

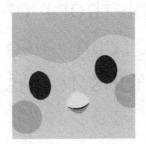

Finch Self Care Pet: Take care of your pet by completing your own self care!

```
Q S V P X M L W I W
Z U Z K K X B C I Y
Y S I I I Y B Y C L
O D C E O Y R H S H
G E A P T X E B T G
A I L M E K A Q R B
K Q M M B R T C E W
W V D C D Z H S T M
P E A C E Q E E C H
J L O J V X A H H J
```

1. Yoga
2. Breathe
3. Stretch
4. Calm
5. Quiet
6. Peace

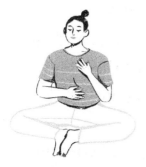

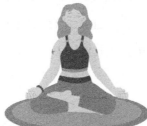

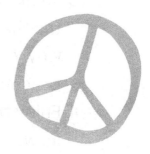

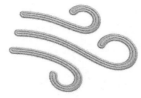

If you can have someone read this outloud, it will certainly make it more relaxing. However if you find yourself alone, read the steps below to yourself and try and relax your body and spirit.

1. Imagine yourself in a comfortable area, the place you feel most at peace. Maybe it is a beach, a riverside cottage, or your own comfy recliner.
2. Focus on your breath, hold for three to five seconds and let your body relax.
3. Think about the sounds, the smells and all the things that relax you about this place, why you enjoy it and why it is your peaceful place.
4. Enjoy the calm moments you find yourself in, whether it's just a moment or a nap worthy experience!

Virtual Travel?

Yes! It exists! If your loved one has experiences they would like to see, it's worth looking to see about virtual travel experiences! For example if they are a lover of art, you can virtually visit a Vincent Van Gogh museum!

His most famous masterpiece, The Starry Night, is at the MoMA in New York City. But there is this pretty cool VR/360 video that lets you immerse into the painting. It is worth checking out!

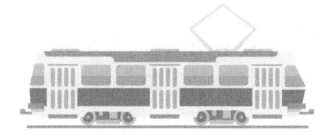

The link below will show you a whole list of amazing virtual experiences!

https://www.globotreks.com/tips/best-virtual-tours-world/

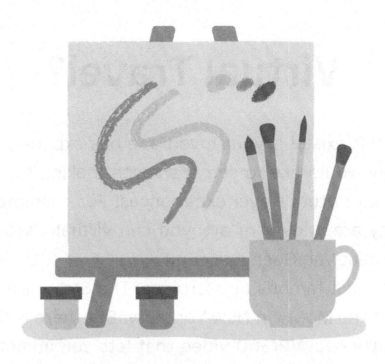

Virtual Museums

The British Museum

https://artsandculture.google.com
/partner/the-british-museum

Mexico City Museum

https://artsandculture.google.com/asset/the-national-
museum-of-anthropology-mexico-city-ziko-van-dijk-
wikimedia-commons/bAGSHRdlzSRcdQ?hl=en

Staatliche Museum

https://artsandculture.google.com/p
artner/pergamonmuseum-
staatliche-museen-zu-berlin?hl=en

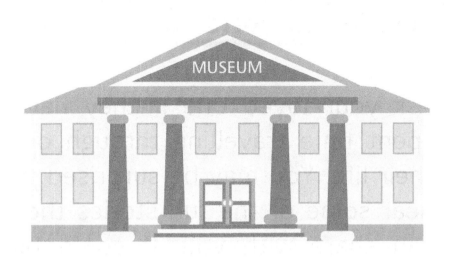

Try Local Museums

Fun times can be had in your own city! Try looking for the nearest local museum, you might find some very interesting information about the place you live. Your loved one also might have some fun memories associated with the cities history!

Where in the world have you been?

Ask your loved one if they have spent time travelling through out their life. You may be surprised to hear some of the fun stories they can share with you. It could be backpacking through countries or simply a good family camping trip - either way this can help trigger happy memories and reboot the joy that they experienced many years ago.

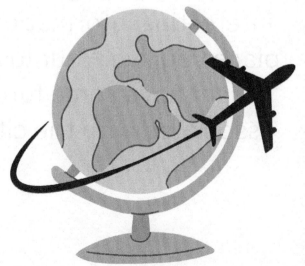

chapter ten

Fond memories and memory
making together

As a caregiver, you have the ability to create cherished memories through simple and regular activities. Whether it's watching a favorite game show on TV or creating a photo album, you play a vital role in providing comfort and joy to your loved one. By engaging in everyday activities and events, you can make a lasting impact on their overall well-being and happiness. Take time to plan meaningful activities that your loved one can enjoy and look back on with fondness. Your efforts will not go unnoticed and will lead to a stronger bond between you and your loved one.

Milestones in life are fondly remembered. It's important to reminisce about these wonderful moments as they help bring joy to everyone! Share some find memories together as often as possible!

Do you have any fond memories of birthdays?

Do you have any fond memories of vacations?

Do you have any fond memories of your career?

Do you have any fond memories of your friends?

You can create a simple slideshow for your loved ones by adding pictures to your phone or computer and having them click through, or if you're more computer savvy you can create a PowerPoint presentation of a beautiful set of photos. Either way, you can entice memories and trigger happy emotions with pictures. These slideshows are a great way to improve the mood and help boost memories that your loved one truly enjoyed.

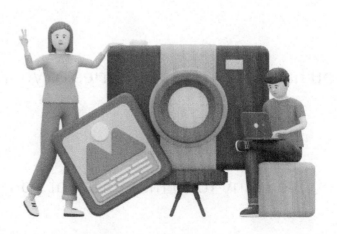

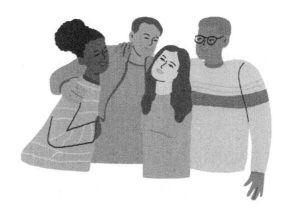

What is your favorite holiday?

What decade was your favorite?

Who is your longest friend?

What hobbies did you have as a kid?

Keeping old birthday or holiday cards is a great way to trigger happy memories. Being able to look back on these moments and reflect on the past is a positive experience and brings a lot of people joy in their later years. If you haven't started already, start keeping as many reminders of the past as you can find!

Another way to keep up on this would be to find a penpal! You may be able to connect with a local community center or find a safe hub online in which you can share letters and birthday cards!

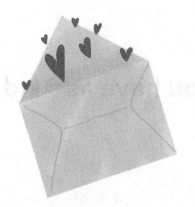

To My Dearest...

Have a look through the prompts below and use one that stands out to you to help start writing!

1. A Letter to:

- Loved Ones
- Old Friends
- A Lost Love
- A Pen Pal
- Someone Missed

2. A Letter about:

- Favorite Places or Activities
- Memorable Trips
- Cherished Moments
- Past Adventures
- Hopes and Dreams

(Use the following page to write out your Letter)

Use the space provided below to write out your letter!

_____

_____

_____

_____

_____

_____

_____

_____

_____

_____

_____

_____

Let's make a scrapbook

- Gather your favourite pictures
- Gather a batch of stickers
- Gather some colored markers
- Paste your photos, add your stickers
- Write some of the memories that were triggered!

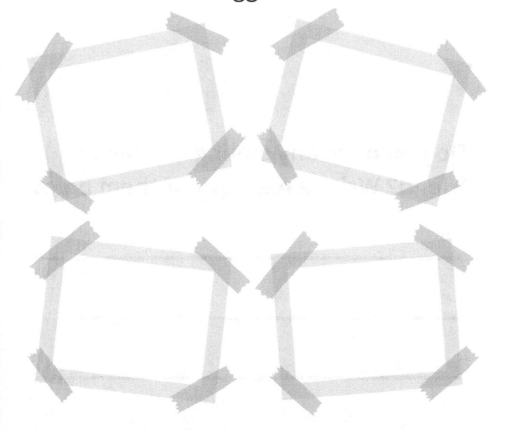

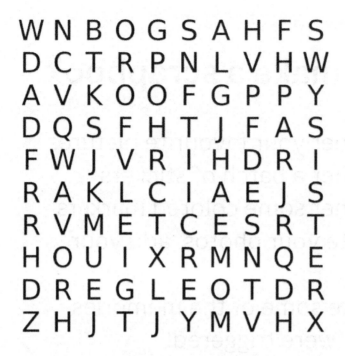

```
W N B O G S A H F S
D C T R P N L V H W
A V K O O F G P P Y
D Q S F H T J F A S
F W J V R I H D R I
R A K L C I A E J S
R V M E T C E S R T
H O U I X R M N Q E
D R E G L E O T D R
Z H J T J Y M V H X
```

1. Brother
2. Sister
3. Mom
4. Dad
5. Friend
6. Family

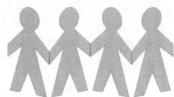

Do you have any siblings? A best friend? Write a memory of them below!

_____

_____

_____

additional resources
and fun ideas

Engaging in activity books and games is a wonderful method to enhance memory skills while forging memories together. These activities instill a sense of fun and entertainment while encouraging cognitive growth. Moreover, by participating as a team, individuals become more inclined to work together and better their communication, problem solving, and critical thinking abilities. As such, investing in such pursuits helps promote familial and social bonds while enhancing cognitive abilities.

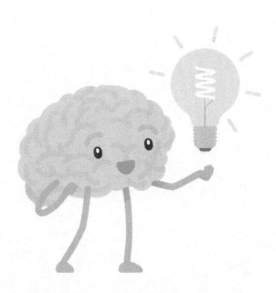

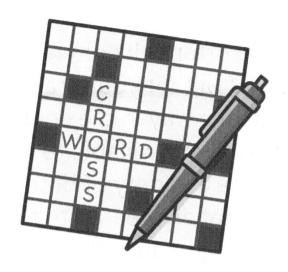

Participating in memory-enhancing activities such as puzzles, games, and mental exercises has numerous benefits for the brain. These activities can increase the usage of neurons, creating new pathways that help the brain store and retrieve memories. Experts recommend engaging in such activities regularly to maintain cognitive function and prevent or delay age-related decline. By keeping the brain active, individuals can improve their memory, attention, and problem-solving abilities, enhancing their overall quality of life.

While we often tell our children "too much TV will rot your brain", we've come a long way in the content that has become available to people. There are a variety of different TV shows that are geared to teaching you things and playing games!

You can find games on TV, documentaries and even music channels to help stimulate your loved ones brain any time of day!

National Geographic has a few videos on YouTube that you can actually utilize at home. There are a few examples below of the videos that they have created for public viewing. There's a lot of fun videos and interactive clips - searching YouTube is an excellent start!

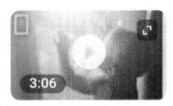

What Do You See? | Brain Games
YouTube · National Geographic
Jun 23, 2015

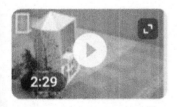

Take the Money... and Run? | Brain Games
YouTube · National Geographic
Jan 15, 2014

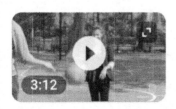

The Power of Positivity | Brain Games
YouTube · National Geographic
Jun 22, 2015

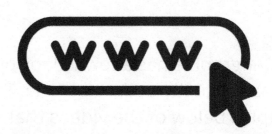

Below you will find websites that you can find worksheets, activities and games that are for all comprehension levels. These are fun for the entire family!

https://www.education.com/

https://www.theteacherscorner.net/

https://www.turtlediary.com/

https://dailycaring.com/

Family Caregiver Alliance – Dementia Caregiver Resources

The Family Caregiver Alliance provides an abundance of resources for caregivers providing care to people with a variety of health conditions and disabilities. The Dementia Caregiver Resources section is a trove of helpful guides, tips sheets, and caregiver stories to help caregivers navigate the journey of caring for a loved one with dementia.

https://www.caregiver.org/caregiver-resources/health-conditions/dementia/

The Alzheimer's Association's 24/7 Helpline

When you're in the midst of a crisis, dementia caregivers can call the Alzheimer's Association's Helpline 24 hours a day, 7 days per week to talk to master's-level clinicians and specialists. This helpline offers crisis guidance, decision support, education, information on local programs and services, information on financial and legal resources, treatment options, and care decisions. There's also a live chat option available from 7:00 a.m. to 7:00 p.m., Monday through Friday. The Alzheimer's Association offers plenty of downloadable resources, too, covering many questions and concerns dementia caregivers face.

Caregivers are truly remarkable individuals who not only provide care but also offer love and support to those in need. They dedicate their time, energy and attention to ensure the wellbeing of their loved ones. These selfless individuals deserve our utmost respect and appreciation for the vital role they play in our society. They exhibit immense strength, compassion and empathy, making a significant difference in the lives of those they care for. We should acknowledge and honor these caregivers for their invaluable contributions to our families and communities.

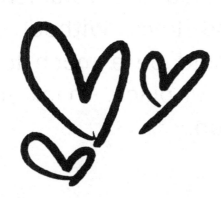

THANK YOU

We express our sincere gratitude to caregivers who support individuals with cognitive disabilities. Your selflessness, compassion, and unwavering commitment to their wellbeing is truly remarkable. Your dedication to enhancing the lives of those in need is a testament to your grace and love. Without you, the world would be a much less bright and hopeful place. Thank you for all that you do.

References

https://www.amazon.com/Dementia-Activity-Studio/e/B07SX128DW
TITLE: Dementia Activity Studio: books, biography, latest update

https://www.mcgill.ca/medsimcentre/files/medsimcentre/dementia_activity_booklet_english_pages_1-55.pdf
TITLE: Created by Occupational Therapy Students For caregivers

https://www.nia.nih.gov/research/alzheimers-dementia-outreach-recruitment-engagement-resources/activity-books-individuals
TITLE: Activity Books for Individuals Experiencing Memory Loss Alzheimer's Disease Center Contact

nia.nih.gov - An official website of the National Institutes of Health Accessibility statement FOIA requests No FEAR Act data Office of the Inspector General Performance reports Vulnerability disclosure policy Policies and notices USA.gov

https://education.com/ - All level reading and writing actitivies on a free or purchase basis

Acknowledging memory changes in a friend or family member can be difficult. It's not uncommon to claim it's a normal part of aging as a way to minimize what it may mean to your family. In truth, we know that serious memory loss is not a normal part of aging, and none of us should ignore or downplay it.

If you or someone you love needs support, please reach out to the Family Caregiver Alliance, one of the best online resource centres for caregivers of people living with dementia.

Are you looking to delve deeper into the world of dementia caregiving? To further equip yourself with practical knowledge, insights, and tools that can make your caregiving journey smoother? We're delighted to introduce the "Dementia Caregiver's Practical Guide: Manage Stress, Avoid Burnout, Find Hope, and Build Resilience" — a comprehensive resource tailored for caregivers like you.

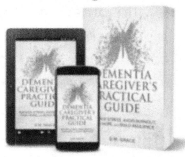

Whether you're in the initial stages of understanding dementia or have been on this journey for some time, this guide promises valuable insights, techniques, and real-life solutions to the challenges faced by caregivers.

How to Access: We've incorporated a QR code on the next page for your convenience. Scan it with your smartphone or tablet, and it will lead you directly to the purchasing page for the "Dementia Caregiver's Practical Guide: Manage Stress, Avoid Burnout, Find Hope, and Build Resilience."
This seamless process ensures that the next step in your caregiving resource journey is just a scan away.

I genuinely believe in empowering caregivers with the best knowledge and support available. This guide is a testament to that belief. May it serve as a beacon of hope, clarity, and practical wisdom in your
journey with your loved one.

Your Feedback Matters to Me!

I hope you are finding value in this journal. Your feedback is crucial to help me and others in this community of caregivers make informed choices. I would be deeply appreciative if you could spare a few minutes to share your thoughts and experiences on Amazon.

How to Leave a Review:

Scan the QR code below using your
smartphone or tablet's camera. This will direct you straight to the review page on Amazon. Share your honest feedback and rate the journal as per your experience.

Your insights not only help future readers/customers but also guide us in our mission to constantly improve and serve you better.

Thank you for your trust, time, and support!

Made in the USA
Monee, IL
25 January 2024

52334538R00083